Dr. Frank N. Scott

THE
CANCER
BLUEPRINT.

A groundbreaking and innovative comprehension of the history of medicine.

CONTENTS

CONTENTS

INTRODUCTION.

CHAPTER ONE
WHAT IS CANCER?
WHAT IS A TUMOR?
WHAT CAUSES CANCER?
TYPES OF CANCER.
CARCINOMAS
SARCOMA
LEUKEMIA
LYMPHOMA AND MYELOMA
BRAIN AND SPINAL CORD CANCER
HISTORY OF CANCER.
CARCINOGENS.
HOW CARCINOGENS CAUSE CANCER.
10 COMMON CARCINOGENS IN OUR DAILY
LIFE.

CHAPTER TWO
    CANCER AND GENETICS
    GENETIC MUTATION
    MUTATION AND CANCER

CHAPTER THREE
    CANCER STAGING
    WHEN IS CANCER STAGING DONE?
    WHAT IS THE TNM STAGING SYSTEM FOR CANCER?
        OTHER FACTORS USED IN CANCER STAGING
    CANCER STAGE GROUPING
    CANCER RESTAGING.

CHAPTER FOUR
    TREATMENT AND IMPLICATION
        BIOMARKER TESTING FOR CANCER.

INTRODUCTION.

Cancer is a condition characterized by the uncontrolled growth and spread of cells in the body. Normally, cells divide and multiply to replace damaged or dying cells. However, cancer cells grow uncontrollably due to DNA damage, which can be inherited or caused by environmental factors such as tobacco or UV rays. Cancer can occur in any part of the body and is often diagnosed through symptoms such as lumps, pain, or changes in bodily functions.

One of the main differences between cancer cells and normal cells is how they grow and interact with other cells. Normal cells stop growing when there are enough cells, whereas cancer cells continue to grow and divide uncontrollably. Cancer cells do not interact with other cells and do not respond to signals from other cells like normal cells do. Additionally, normal cells repair themselves or die to maintain balance, whereas cancer cells do not self-repair or undergo apoptosis.

Genetic changes play a significant role in the development of cancer. DNA damage caused by factors such as errors in cell division, exposure to environmental substances, or inherited mutations can lead to the development of cancer. As the body's ability to kill damaged cells decreases with age, the risk of developing cancer increases with age.

Metastasis occurs when cancer cells travel to other parts of the body and form new tumors. The name and type of initial cancer also apply to metastatic cancer. Cancer treatment often involves a combination of surgery, radiation therapy, chemotherapy, and targeted therapy. Regular cancer screenings can help detect cancer early, improving the chances of successful treatment.

CHAPTER ONE

WHAT IS CANCER?

Cancer refers to a diverse group of diseases that can originate from any part of the body, in which abnormal cells grow uncontrollably, infiltrate surrounding tissues, and sometimes spread to other organs through metastasis. This process is a leading cause of death from cancer. Other names for cancer include malignant tumors and neoplasms.

Globally, cancer is responsible for a significant proportion of deaths, with an estimated 9.6 million deaths in 2018, making it the second leading cause of death. The most common types of cancer vary between genders, with lung, prostate, colorectal, stomach, and liver cancer being the most common in men, and breast, colorectal, lung, cervical, and thyroid cancer being the most common in women.

The burden of cancer is increasing worldwide, and it has a substantial impact on individuals, families, communities, and healthcare systems, with low- and middle-income countries being the least equipped to manage this burden. Many cancer patients worldwide do not have timely access to high-quality diagnosis and treatment. However, in countries with strong healthcare systems, the survival rates of several types of cancer have improved due to accessible early detection, quality treatment, and survivorship care.

Your body is composed of trillions of cells that typically grow and divide as needed throughout your life. Under normal circumstances, abnormal or old cells die off. However, cancer occurs when there is a problem in this process, and your cells continue to multiply and old or abnormal cells do not die when they should. This leads to the formation of cancerous cells that can grow uncontrollably and crowd out normal cells, which can affect the functioning of your body.

It is important to note that cancer is not just one disease, but rather a collection of many different types of cancers. Cancer can originate from any part of the body, and the type of cancer is usually named after the location where it started. For instance, breast cancer that develops in the breast is still referred to as breast cancer even if it spreads to other parts of the body.

There are two primary categories of cancer: hematologic (blood) cancers and solid tumor cancers. Hematologic cancers refer to cancers that develop in blood cells, such as leukemia, lymphoma, and multiple myeloma. On the other hand, solid tumor cancers can occur in any of the other organs or tissues in the body, with the most common types being breast, prostate, lung, and colorectal cancers.

These cancers share some similarities but can differ in terms of how they grow, spread, and respond to treatment. Some types of cancer can spread quickly, while others grow more slowly or tend to stay where they started.

The cancer treatment varies depending on the type and stage of the cancer. Some cancers can be treated with surgery, while others may respond better to drugs like chemotherapy. In some cases, a combination of two or more treatments is required to achieve the best results. While cancer can be a serious disease, it is important to remember that many people can be successfully treated for cancer, and an increasing number of people can lead full lives after cancer treatment.

WHAT IS A TUMOR?

A tumor is a mass or growth that can be present in different parts of the body. While some lumps are cancerous, many others are not. If the growth is not cancerous, it is referred to as benign. However, if the lump is cancerous, it is called malignant.

What sets cancer apart from benign tumors is its ability to spread to other parts of the body. When cancer cells grow uncontrollably, they can break away from the site where they started and travel to other parts of the body through the bloodstream or lymphatic system. Once cancer cells reach other organs or tissues, they can interfere with the normal functions of those areas, leading to a range of problems.

WHAT CAUSES CANCER?

Cancer cells develop as a result of multiple changes in their genes, and these changes can have various causes. For example, unhealthy lifestyle habits, such as smoking, excessive alcohol consumption, and poor diet, can contribute to the development of cancer. In some cases, people may inherit genes from their parents that increase their risk of developing certain types of cancer. Exposure to cancer-causing agents in the environment, such as radiation, pollution, and certain chemicals, can also play a role in the development of cancer. However, in many cases, there is no obvious cause for the development of cancer.

TYPES OF CANCER.

Cancer can be categorized based on the type of cell that it originates from. There are five major categories of cancer, which include:

Carcinoma: This type of cancer starts in the epithelial cells that form the lining of organs or tissues in the body. Carcinomas can invade surrounding tissues and organs and spread to other parts of the body. The most common forms of carcinoma are breast, prostate, lung, and colon cancer.

Sarcoma: Sarcoma is a type of cancer that develops in the bone or soft tissue, such as fat, muscle, blood vessels, nerves, and other connective tissues that surround and support organs. Some common forms of sarcoma include leiomyosarcoma, liposarcoma, and osteosarcoma.

Lymphoma and Myeloma: Lymphoma and myeloma are cancers that originate in the immune system cells. Lymphoma is a cancer of the lymphatic system, which is present throughout the body, while myeloma begins in the plasma cells, a type of white blood cell responsible for producing antibodies that help fight infections.

Leukemia: Leukemia is a cancer of the bone marrow and white blood cells. There are several subtypes of leukemia, including lymphocytic leukemia and chronic lymphocytic leukemia.

Brain and spinal cord cancers: These types of cancer, also known as central nervous system cancers, can be benign or malignant. Some common types of brain and spinal cord cancers include glioma, astrocytoma, and medulloblastoma.

Cancer can have various causes, including lifestyle habits, genetic factors, and exposure to cancer-causing agents in the environment. However, in some cases, the cause of cancer may not be apparent. It's important to note that not all lumps or growths are cancerous, and benign tumors do not spread to other parts of the body, unlike malignant tumors. Cancer treatment may vary depending on the type of cancer and its stage and can include surgery, chemotherapy, radiation therapy, and immunotherapy, among other approaches.

CARCINOMAS

Carcinomas are a type of cancer that originates in the epithelial tissues of the body, which cover the surface of the body, line the organs, and also line the body cavities. This means that carcinomas can arise from various tissues in the body, including the skin and the organs of the digestive system, chest cavity, and abdominal cavity. Carcinomas are the most common type of cancer, accounting for about 85% of all cancers in the UK.

Several types of epithelial cells can develop into different subtypes of carcinoma. Squamous cell carcinoma is a type of cancer that arises from the flat, scale-like cells that make up the epithelial tissue in the skin and the lining of some organs such as the esophagus and lungs. Adenocarcinoma, on the other hand, starts in glandular cells that produce fluids such as mucus and can be found in organs such as the breast, pancreas, and prostate. Transitional cell carcinoma arises from the transitional cells that line the bladder, while basal cell carcinoma is a type of skin cancer that originates from the basal cells that are located in the lowest layer of the epidermis.

SARCOMA

To put it in simpler terms, sarcomas are a type of cancer that develops in the body's supporting tissues, which are called connective tissues. These tissues provide structure and support to organs, bones, and muscles. Sarcomas are not as common as carcinomas and make up only a small percentage of cancer diagnoses. There are two main types of sarcomas: bone sarcomas and soft tissue sarcomas. Bone sarcomas originate from the cells of bones, while soft tissue sarcomas start in the non-bony parts of the body's connective tissues, such as muscles, cartilage, tendons, and fibrous tissue. Sarcomas that start in cartilage are called chondrosarcomas and develop from cartilage cells known as chondroblasts. Sarcomas that develop in muscle cells are called rhabdomyosarcomas or leiomyosarcomas. It's essential to note that sarcomas are rare and account for only a small percentage of cancer diagnoses.

LEUKEMIA

Leukemia is a type of cancer that affects the white blood cells, which are important components of the body's immune system. In leukemia, the bone marrow produces too many white blood cells, but they do not mature properly and are unable to function effectively. These abnormal cells then accumulate in the blood, where they can interfere with the normal functions of the body. Leukemia is not very common, accounting for only 3% of all cancer cases. However, it is the most common type of cancer in children.

There are several subtypes of leukemia, including lymphocytic leukemia and chronic lymphocytic leukemia. These subtypes are classified based on the type of white blood cell affected and the rate of progression of the disease. Leukemia can cause a variety of symptoms, including fatigue, weakness, fever, weight loss, and frequent infections. Treatment options for leukemia depend on the type and stage of the disease but may include chemotherapy, radiation therapy, stem cell transplantation, and targeted therapy. Early diagnosis and treatment are important for improving the chances of a successful outcome.

LYMPHOMA AND MYELOMA

Lymphomas and myeloma are types of cancer that affect the lymphatic system. The lymphatic system is responsible for filtering body fluids and fighting off infections. Lymphoma is a type of cancer that starts in the lymphatic system and can occur anywhere in the body as the lymphatic system runs throughout the entire body. Abnormal lymphocytes, a type of white blood cell, start to divide abnormally and don't mature, making them ineffective in fighting off infections. The abnormal cells accumulate in the lymph nodes or other areas, and tumors can form. Lymphomas account for approximately 5% of all cancer cases in the UK.

Myeloma is a type of cancer that starts in the plasma cells, a type of white blood cell produced in the bone marrow that produces antibodies to fight infections. Abnormal plasma cells can multiply uncontrollably and produce an ineffective type of antibody that cannot fight off infections. Myeloma is relatively rare, accounting for only 1% of all cancer cases in the UK.

BRAIN AND SPINAL CORD CANCER

Cancer that affects the brain or spinal cord originates from the abnormal growth of cells in these organs. The brain is responsible for controlling the body's functions by sending electrical signals through nerve fibers that run out of the brain and join together to form the spinal cord. Together, these two structures form the central nervous system.

The brain is made up of billions of nerve cells called neurons, which communicate with each other to coordinate the body's activities. The neurons are supported by glial cells, a type of connective tissue cell that surrounds and protects the nerve cells.

The most common type of brain tumor is glioma, which develops from glial cells. Some brain and spinal cord tumors are benign, meaning they grow slowly and do not spread to other parts of the body. Others are malignant or cancerous and tend to grow and spread to other parts of the brain or spinal cord. Brain and spinal cord tumors are relatively uncommon, accounting for only 3% of all cancer cases in the UK. Nonetheless, they can have serious consequences due to their impact on the central nervous system, which controls the body's functions. Early detection and treatment are essential for improving the chances of successful treatment and recovery.

HISTORY OF CANCER.

Cancer is a disease that can be traced back to prehistoric times, with evidence of its existence found in dinosaur fossils that date back over 70 million years. In humans, the earliest known case of cancer was documented in an Egyptian man who lived around 3,000 years ago.

Over time, cancer has become more prevalent due to several factors, including longer life expectancy and increased exposure to carcinogens in our environment. While cancer was known to ancient civilizations such as the Egyptians, it wasn't until much later that medical treatments for the disease were developed. The first written evidence of cancer comes from ancient Egyptian manuscripts dating back to between 1500 and 1600 BCE. These manuscripts describe a variety of treatments, ranging from pharmacological and surgical to magical, but the Egyptians believed that the disease was incurable and blamed it on the gods.

The origin of the term "cancer" can be traced back to around 400 BCE, when Hippocrates, an ancient Greek physician considered the "Father of

Medicine", used the terms karkino and carcinoma to describe a type of disease caused by an imbalance of the body's four humors: blood, yellow bile, phlegm, and black bile. Hippocrates and his followers, known as the physicians of the Hippocratic school, were able to distinguish between benign and malignant tumors and had some knowledge about the invasive nature of the disease.

During the Byzantine Empire, medical researchers discovered the presence of lymph nodes in the chests of women with breast cancer and used poppyseed extracts to alleviate the pain. However, their attempts to remove tumors were not very successful.

In Europe between 500 and 1500 CE, various treatments for cancer were developed, including the removal and cauterization of small tumors, and the use of caustic arsenic pastes, diets, crab powder, and amulets for larger tumors. With the advent of autopsies from 1500 CE, knowledge of internal cancers grew, although, before that time, only external tumors could be studied.

In the 17th century, several significant advances were made in cancer research, including the invention of the lens microscope, which made it possible to see blood cells and bacteria, and the first successful mastectomies.

In recent times, there has been significant progress in understanding the disease, including the recognition of its genetic origins. This knowledge has enabled the development of personalized treatment plans for patients, tailored to their specific genetic makeup.

However, while cancer itself has not changed, the incidence of each type of tumor has, with lung cancer now being the most commonly diagnosed and deadliest form, despite being a rare disease before 1900.

CARCINOGENS.

Carcinogens refer to substances or exposures that can trigger the development of cancer in humans. These may include a wide range of chemical and physical agents, such as toxic chemicals commonly found in homes and workplaces, radiation from various sources like sunlight, medical equipment, or industrial processes, smoke from tobacco products, and even some viruses and medications.

Identifying carcinogens is a crucial step in preventing and controlling cancer. Researchers use various methods to determine if a substance is a carcinogen or not, including animal and human studies, lab experiments, and observational studies. Once a substance has been identified as a potential carcinogen, regulatory agencies take steps to limit or ban its use to protect public health.

While it's impossible to avoid exposure to all carcinogens, taking steps to reduce your exposure can significantly lower your risk of developing cancer. Simple lifestyle changes, such as quitting smoking, reducing alcohol consumption, and limiting sun exposure can go a long way in protecting yourself from cancer. Avoiding environmental toxins, using protective gear in workplaces, and following safe handling procedures for chemicals can also help minimize exposure.

In conclusion, understanding carcinogens and how to limit exposure is essential to protecting your health and preventing cancer. With the right knowledge and precautions, you can significantly reduce your risk of developing cancer and live a healthier life.

HOW CARCINOGENS CAUSE CANCER.

Carcinogens are substances or agents that can cause cancer by harming the genetic material or DNA within your cells. When a carcinogen enters your body, it can interact with your DNA in different ways. Some carcinogens can directly damage the DNA strands, resulting in genetic mutations that alter the normal functioning of the cells. These mutations can affect genes that control cell growth, division, and death, leading to abnormal cell growth and the formation of cancerous tumors.

In other cases, carcinogens may trigger inflammation in the cells, leading to an increased rate of cell division. This increased cell division can also increase the likelihood of DNA mutations occurring. These mutations can then further alter the cell's function and behavior, leading to the development of cancer.

It's important to note that not all exposures to carcinogens will result in cancer. The effects of carcinogens can vary depending on factors such as the duration and intensity of exposure, as well as an

21

individual's genetic susceptibility. However, it's crucial to limit your exposure to known carcinogens to reduce your risk of developing cancer.

10 COMMON CARCINOGENS IN OUR DAILY LIFE.

These 10 items are common examples of carcinogens or substances that can cause cancer. One way that these substances can contribute to cancer is by damaging DNA, which carries genetic information in your cells. Here are some tips to reduce your exposure to these carcinogens:

Browned and crispy foods - Cooking starchy foods in a way that causes them to brown could create carcinogens, such as acrylamide. To reduce your exposure, try frying potatoes to a lighter yellow color or not over-toasting your bread.

Sunlight - Too much exposure to sunlight and ultraviolet rays (UV) increases skin cancer risk. Protect yourself by wearing hats and protective clothing, applying sunscreen, and avoiding the midday sun.

Processed meat - Processed meats are preserved with chemicals like nitrates and nitrites, and cooked at high heat, which creates polycyclic amines and heterocyclic amines. Try avoiding processed meats, decrease your portion size, and replace deli meat with fish or tofu.

Tobacco - Tobacco use is the leading cause of cancer and can lead to many different types of cancer, including lung, throat, esophageal, colon, and bladder cancer. Talk with your healthcare provider about getting the help you or your loved ones need to quit smoking.

Radon - Radon is a silent and odorless gas that can increase lung cancer risk. Test your level and take steps to mitigate it such as by improving airflow and ventilation.

Air pollution - Polluted air and exhaust from vehicles can increase cancer risk, particularly lung and breast cancer. Avoid exposure to engine exhaust for too long and consider wearing a mask or using an air filter to help remove some particles from the air you breathe.

Bisphenol A - BPA is a chemical found in many products and can mimic the hormone estrogen, potentially increasing the risk of cancer such as prostate or breast cancer. Avoid products with BPA by checking the label.

Alcohol - Alcohol consumption has been linked to different types of cancer including liver, breast, and esophageal cancer. Limit your consumption to the recommended amount of one drink a day for women and two for men.

Formaldehyde - Formaldehyde is a chemical present in many household items and is also produced while using gas stoves. Check the formaldehyde level of products before putting in new furniture or products in your home and make sure you have ventilation.

Polychlorinated biphenyls - PCBs are man-made chemicals that have been used in electrical equipment and plastics. Although they are no longer produced, they are still present in soil and water, and in foods like meat, fish, and dairy.

CHAPTER TWO

CANCER AND GENETICS

Genes are the basic units of heredity and are found in the DNA of every cell in your body. They play a vital role in controlling how cells function, including their rate of growth, frequency of division, and lifespan. There are approximately 30,000 different genes in each cell, and they are located on thread-like structures called chromosomes.

Humans have 46 chromosomes, arranged in two sets of 23. One of the sets is from the mother, and the other is from the father. The chromosomes determine physical characteristics, including sex, which is determined by one chromosome pair, and other traits, which are determined by the other 22 pairs.

Genes work by producing proteins, which have specific functions and act as messengers for the cell. For each gene to make its specific protein, it must have the correct instructions. When one or more genes in a cell mutate, they create abnormal proteins that provide different information than normal proteins. This can cause cells to multiply uncontrollably and become cancerous, leading to the development of cancer.

In summary, genes are the building blocks of heredity, and they play a critical role in controlling cell functions. Mutations in genes can lead to the development of cancer by causing cells to multiply uncontrollably due to the production of abnormal proteins.

GENETIC MUTATION

The genetic makeup of an individual plays a crucial role in determining their risk of developing cancer. Mutations, or changes, in genes can lead to the development of cancer. Two primary types of genetic mutations can cause cancer: acquired mutations and germline mutations.

Acquired mutations are the most common cause of cancer. These mutations occur when genes in a particular cell are damaged during an individual's lifetime. For instance, exposure to harmful substances such as tobacco or ultraviolet (UV) radiation can damage genes in cells, which may then divide and form a tumor. A tumor is an abnormal mass of cells that can be cancerous or non-cancerous. These acquired mutations are not present in every cell of the body, and they cannot be passed down from parents to children. Cancer that develops as a result of acquired mutations is referred to as sporadic cancer.

Several factors can cause acquired mutations, including exposure to tobacco, UV radiation, certain viruses, and advancing age.

Germline mutations are less common than acquired mutations. These mutations occur in the sperm or egg cells and are passed directly from a parent to their child during conception. As the embryo develops into a mature baby, the mutation from the initial sperm or egg cell is copied into all the cells within the body. Since the mutation affects the reproductive cells, it can be passed down from generation to generation. Cancer caused by germline mutations is called inherited cancer and it accounts for approximately 5% to 20% of all cancers.

It is essential to note that not all genetic mutations lead to cancer. Some mutations do not affect an individual's health, while others may even offer protection against certain diseases. Genetic testing can help identify mutations that increase an individual's risk of developing cancer, allowing for proactive measures to be taken to reduce their risk.

MUTATION AND CANCER

Mutations are common and can be beneficial, harmful, or have no effect, depending on where they occur in the gene. The body can usually correct most mutations, and a single mutation is unlikely to cause cancer. Cancer usually develops due to multiple mutations over a person's lifetime, which is why it occurs more frequently in older individuals who have had more opportunities for mutations to accumulate.

There are several types of genes linked to cancer, including tumor suppressor genes, oncogenes, and DNA repair genes. Tumor suppressor genes normally limit cell growth and repair mismatched DNA or control when a cell dies. When they mutate, cells can grow uncontrollably and form tumors. Examples of tumor suppressor genes include BRCA1, BRCA2, and p53 or TP53, which are associated with increased risks of developing various types of cancer.

Oncogenes, on the other hand, turn healthy cells into cancerous ones, and mutations in these genes are not usually inherited. Two common oncogenes are HER2, which controls cancer growth and spread, and the RAS family of genes, which are involved in cell communication pathways, cell growth, and cell death.

DNA repair genes fix mistakes made when DNA is copied and often function as tumor suppressor genes. If these genes have an error, mutations can accumulate and lead to cancer, particularly in tumor suppressor genes or oncogenes. Mutations in DNA repair genes may be inherited or acquired, and examples of inherited mutations include Lynch syndrome and syndromes associated with BRCA1, BRCA2, and p53 genes.

……...

Recent research on breast and colorectal cancers has found that while most cases are sporadic, some are familial. Sporadic breast cancer typically develops later in life, while familial forms can appear much earlier, often before age 40. Inherited mutations in the BRCA1 and BRCA2 genes account for at least half of all familial breast cancer cases, as these genes encode proteins that play a role in DNA damage response pathways. Women with these mutations are at a much higher risk of developing breast cancer and may also be at risk for ovarian tumors. The mutated gene can be passed down from both men and women to their offspring, with carrier daughters at a higher risk of developing breast cancer.

Similarly, two forms of familial colorectal cancer, HNPCC, and FAP have also been linked to predisposing mutations in specific genes. Individuals with HNPCC have inherited mutations in their DNA mismatch repair genes, while those with FAP carry inherited mutations in their APC genes, which function as tumor suppressor. In both cases, the combination of inherited and somatic mutations leads to a high lifetime risk of developing colorectal cancer.

Despite the majority of cancer cases being sporadic, all cancers are genetic diseases. Research suggests that cancer arises from successive mutations that work together to disrupt normal cell growth, facilitate blood supply to tumors, and enable metastasis.

CHAPTER THREE

CANCER STAGING

Staging a cancer is an important process that involves describing its location, size, and how far it has grown into nearby tissues, as well as if it has advanced to other parts of the body or lymph nodes. It is usually done before starting any treatment and may not be completed until all the necessary tests have been conducted. The stage of a cancer is an essential factor in determining the most effective treatment plan, including the type of surgery and whether chemotherapy or radiation therapy will be necessary.

Doctors can use staging to determine the chances of cancer recurrence or spread after treatment and forecast the prognosis or the chance of recovery. Additionally, staging helps determine which clinical trials may be open to the patient and how well a treatment worked. The entire healthcare team can also use staging to discuss the diagnosis uniformly, which is beneficial for the patient.

Staging is usually done using physical exams, imaging scans, and other tests. The process may involve different stages, depending on the type of cancer. For instance, breast cancer has four stages while colon cancer has five stages. Doctors use different methods to determine the stage of cancer, including biopsy, blood tests, X-rays, and MRI scans. The combination of these methods can provide a more accurate picture of the cancer stage and help doctors develop a tailored treatment plan. In conclusion, cancer staging is a crucial step in diagnosing and treating cancer. It provides valuable information about the location, size, and spread of the cancer, which helps doctors determine the most effective treatment plan. Understanding the cancer stage can also help patients and their families prepare for the treatment and make informed decisions about their health.

WHEN IS CANCER STAGING DONE?

Cancer staging is a critical aspect of cancer diagnosis and treatment. Staging determines the extent to which cancer has spread, which guides the selection of appropriate treatment options and helps predict a person's prognosis. Staging is typically done at different points during a person's medical care, and the TNM system is used to categorize cancer based on the tumor, lymph nodes, and metastasis.

Clinical staging is the first stage of cancer staging and is done before any treatment begins. Your doctor will conduct a physical exam, review your medical history, and perform imaging, scans, and diagnostic tests. They will also analyze the biopsy results of any tissue, lymph nodes, or cancer. The goal of clinical staging is to help you and your doctor plan the initial steps of your treatment. A small "c" is used to indicate clinical staging before the TNM category.

Pathological staging, on the other hand, is based on the same information as clinical staging, but it includes any new information gathered during surgery, particularly if surgery was the first treatment for the type of cancer. A small "p" is used to indicate pathological staging before the TNM category.

Post-therapy staging is used when surgery is not the first treatment option. Instead, treatments like radiation therapy or drug treatments like chemotherapy, immunotherapy, or hormone therapy are given before surgery. These treatments may be used to shrink the tumor and make surgery more manageable. Additionally, post-therapy staging can help doctors learn how well treatments work for the type of cancer and plan further treatment. A "y" is used to indicate post-therapy staging before the TNM category.

When doctors determine the stage of a specific type of cancer using the TNM system, clinical staging is always the first step. After the surgical operation or initial treatments before surgery, pathological staging and post-therapy staging should also be used. While clinical staging is essential for planning initial treatment, pathological staging, and post-therapy staging provide more information that can help the healthcare team understand a person's prognosis. Knowing the cancer's stage is critical for developing an effective treatment plan that can help improve a person's quality of life and chances of survival.

WHAT IS THE TNM STAGING SYSTEM FOR CANCER?

The TNM staging system is commonly used by doctors to stage most types of cancer. This system is based on the three key factors that describe the tumor, the lymph nodes, and the presence of metastases. Each letter and number provides valuable information about the type of cancer, and the definitions for each category vary depending on the type of cancer. It is important to understand the specific staging information for each type of cancer.

The T category describes the size, location, and spread of the primary tumor. The letter T, followed by a number or combination of other letters provides additional details about the tumor. The TX category shows that there is no information about the tumor. T0 means there is no evidence of a tumor, while Tis refers to a tumor "in situ", which means that the tumor is only found in the cells where it started growing and has not spread to neighboring tissues. T1-T4 describes the size and location of the tumor on a scale of 1 to 4, with a higher number indicating a larger or more deeply grown tumor. Some types of cancer also have subcategories denoted by a lowercase letter such as "a" or "b" for more detail, and "m" is used to indicate multiple tumors.

The N category describes if cancer has spread to the lymph nodes, which are small organs that help fight infection. The letter N is followed by a number from 0 to 3 that indicates whether there is cancer in the regional lymph nodes, with a higher number indicating more affected nodes. Lymph nodes in other parts of the body are included in the "M" category.

The M category describes whether a specific type of cancer has spread to other parts of the body. M0 means that there is no evidence of metastasis, while M1 indicates that cancer has spread to other parts of the body. Understanding the TNM staging system and the specific information for each category can help doctors develop an effective treatment plan and provide patients with information about their prognosis.

OTHER FACTORS USED IN CANCER STAGING

In some types of cancer, the stage can include factors beyond the TNM categories. These factors are grade, biomarkers, and tumor genetics. The grade of cancer is determined by comparing cancer cells to healthy cells under a microscope. If cancer looks similar to healthy tissue, it is called a low-grade tumor. If cancer looks very different, it is called a high-grade tumor. Cancer's grade can help predict how quickly it will spread. Biomarkers are substances found at higher levels than normal in cancer or the bodily fluids of people with cancer. Biomarkers can help determine the likelihood of cancer spreading and assist doctors in choosing the best treatment. Tumor genetics can help predict if cancer will spread or which treatments will be effective. This information can help doctors create personalized and targeted treatment plans. Each type of cancer has different methods for determining its grade and identifying biomarkers and tumor genetics.

CANCER STAGE GROUPING

When determining the stage of cancer, the TNM categories are used to create a specific stage for each individual. Typically, there are four stages of cancer ranging from stage I (1) to stage IV (4), with some types of cancer also having stage 0 (zero). Although each type of cancer has a specific staging system, here is a general description of cancer stage groupings.

Stage 0 refers to cancer that is in situ, meaning it has not spread beyond its initial location and is often curable. Surgery can often remove the entire tumor.

Stage I usually indicates that cancer has not grown deeply into nearby tissues and has not spread to other parts of the body. This stage is commonly referred to as early-stage cancer.

Stage II and III typically represent cancers that have grown more deeply into nearby tissue and may have also spread to lymph nodes, but not to other parts of the body.

Stage IV means that cancer has spread to other organs or parts of the body, and may also be referred to as advanced or metastatic cancer. The extent of cancer at this stage varies depending on the individual case, and treatment options are often more limited. It is crucial to discuss treatment options with a healthcare provider to determine the best course of action for each case.

CANCER RESTAGING.

When a person is diagnosed with cancer, doctors use the TNM staging system to determine the stage of cancer. The stage is specific to the individual and is used to track the progress of cancer, understand the prognosis, and evaluate how the treatment is affecting the patient. The stage given at the time of diagnosis and initial treatment does not change.

However, if cancer comes back or spreads to other parts of the body, restaging can be done. This is indicated with a small "r" and involves repeating some of the same tests that were done when the cancer was first diagnosed. The results of the tests are used to assign a restage or "r stage" to cancer.

The TNM staging system is mainly used to describe solid tumors like breast, colon, and lung cancers. Other staging systems are used for different types of cancer. For example, childhood cancers are staged using systems specific to that cancer, while blood cancers like leukemia, lymphoma, and multiple myeloma have their staging system. For brain tumors, only the "T" description of the TNM system is used as these tumors do not usually spread outside the brain and spinal cord.

CHAPTER FOUR

TREATMENT AND IMPLICATION

There is a wide range of cancer treatments available, and the specific treatment plan you receive will depend on the type and stage of your cancer. Some individuals may only require a single form of treatment, while others may need a combination of treatments, such as surgery, chemotherapy, and radiation therapy. Facing a cancer diagnosis can be overwhelming, but it is important to talk with your doctor and become informed about the potential treatments you may undergo.

BIOMARKER TESTING FOR CANCER.

One method of determining a cancer treatment plan is through biomarker testing. This involves analyzing genes, proteins, and other substances in the body, known as biomarkers or tumor markers, to gather information about the specific type of cancer. This information can then be used by you and your doctor to choose the most effective cancer treatment. Biomarker testing can also help identify targeted therapies that are specific to your cancer, potentially leading to a more successful treatment outcome.

CHEMOTHERAPY

Chemotherapy, also known as chemo, is a treatment for cancer that involves the use of drugs to kill cancer cells. This treatment is effective because it stops or slows down the growth of cancer cells, which tend to grow and divide quickly. There are two main reasons why chemotherapy is used: to cure cancer or to ease the symptoms associated with it. Depending on the type of cancer, chemotherapy may be used as the sole treatment, or it may be combined with other treatments.

SIDE EFFECTS OF CHEMOTHERAPY

It is important to note that chemotherapy can cause side effects because it not only kills cancer cells but also healthy cells that grow and divide quickly, such as those that line the mouth and intestines and those that cause hair growth. Some common side effects include mouth sores, nausea, hair loss, and fatigue, which is the most common side effect. Fortunately, these side effects usually improve or disappear after treatment is completed. To manage these side effects, patients can prepare by asking for help with driving, meal preparation, and childcare, and planning to rest on the day of and the day after chemotherapy.

HOW CHEMOTHERAPY IS ADMINISTERED

Chemotherapy can be administered in several ways, including orally, intravenously (IV), through injections, intrathecally, intraperitoneally, intra-arterially, and topically. IV chemotherapy is the most common method and involves a thin needle being inserted into a vein in the hand or lower arm, sometimes with the help of a pump. The type of chemotherapy and method of administration will depend on the type of cancer and the individual patient's circumstances. It is important to discuss all treatment options and potential side effects with a healthcare professional to determine the best course of action.

HORMONE THERAPY

Hormone therapy, also known as hormonal therapy, hormone treatment, or endocrine therapy, is a type of cancer treatment that slows down or stops the growth of cancer cells that depend on hormones to grow. There are two main types of hormone therapy: those that block the production of hormones in the body and those that interfere with how hormones work in the body.

Hormone therapy is commonly used to treat breast and prostate cancers, as these types of cancer often depend on hormones to grow. It is usually administered in conjunction with other cancer treatments, and the specific type of hormone therapy that is used depends on the type and stage of cancer, as well as other important factors such as the patient's general health.

SIDE EFFECTS OF HORMONE THERAPY

However, hormone therapy can also cause unwanted side effects as it blocks the body's ability to produce hormones or interferes with the way hormones behave. The specific side effects experienced will depend on the type of hormone therapy administered, as well as individual factors such as the patient's age, gender, and overall health.

For men who receive hormone therapy for prostate cancer, common side effects include hot flashes, reduced sex drive, weakened bones, diarrhea, nausea, enlarged and tender breasts, and fatigue. Women who receive hormone therapy for breast cancer may experience hot flashes, vaginal dryness, changes in menstrual cycles (if they have not yet reached menopause), reduced sex drive, nausea, mood changes, and fatigue. It is important to note that not all patients will experience the same side effects, and some may not experience any at all.

If you are experiencing side effects from hormone therapy, it is important to discuss them with your healthcare team. They may be able to recommend strategies to manage or alleviate your symptoms.

HYPERTHERMIA.

Hyperthermia is a cancer treatment that involves heating body tissue to temperatures as high as 113°F to damage and kill cancer cells while minimizing harm to normal tissue. It is as well known as thermal therapy, thermal ablation, or thermotherapy. Different techniques are used to generate heat, including microwaves, radio waves, lasers, ultrasound, perfusion of heated fluids, and whole-body heating. Hyperthermia is not widely available, but it is used at some centers in combination with other treatments for advanced cancers such as bladder, breast, lung, and brain cancer, among others.

HOW HYPERTHERMIA IS GIVEN.

The doctor numbs the treatment area and inserts small probes with thermometers into the tumor during treatment. Imaging techniques such as CT scans may also be used to ensure the probes are in the correct location. Hyperthermia can be applied to small areas of the body, large areas, or the entire body. Local hyperthermia, which heats a small area, can be achieved using external, intraluminal, or interstitial techniques. Regional hyperthermia, which heats large areas of the body, can be achieved using deep tissue techniques, regional perfusion, or continuous hyperthermic peritoneal perfusion. Whole-body hyperthermia is used in treating cancer that has advanced throughout the body.

SIDE EFFECTS OF HYPERTHERMIA.

Although most healthy tissue is not damaged during hyperthermia if the temperature stays below 111°F, higher temperatures in certain areas may cause burns, blisters, discomfort, or pain. Perfusion techniques may result in swelling, blood clots, bleeding, and other damage to normal tissues in the treated area, but most of these side effects improve after treatment. Whole-body hyperthermia can cause diarrhea, nausea, vomiting, and more serious side effects such as heart and blood vessel problems.

IMMUNOTHERAPY

Immunotherapy is a form of cancer treatment that helps the body's immune system fight cancer. The immune system is composed of white blood cells and lymphatic tissues and organs that protect the body against infections and diseases.
Immunotherapy works by enhancing the immune system's ability to detect and destroy abnormal cells, such as cancer cells. However, cancer cells can sometimes evade destruction by the immune system by having genetic changes that make them less visible, proteins on their surface that turn off immune cells, or by altering normal cells around the tumor.

SIDE EFFECTS OF IMMUNOTHERAPY.
Immunotherapy drugs have been approved to treat
many types of cancer, but they can cause side effects
by mistakenly attacking healthy cells and tissues.

**WAYS OF ADMINISTERING
IMMUNOTHERAPY.**
Different forms of immunotherapy can be given,
including intravenous, oral, topical, and intravesical
administration, depending on the type and stage of
the cancer being treated.

PHOTODYNAMIC THERAPY
Photodynamic therapy, also known as PDT, is a
cancer treatment that involves the use of a
photosensitizing agent, which is activated by light,
to destroy cancer cells. The light source used may be
a laser or LED. Typically, PDT is used to treat a
specific area of the body affected by cancer, making
it a local treatment. PDT has been approved by the
FDA to treat various types of cancer and
precancerous conditions such as actinic keratosis,
basal cell skin cancer, esophageal cancer, and non-
small cell lung cancer.

HOW PDT WORKS

When the photosensitizing agent is exposed to a specific wavelength of light, it creates a form of oxygen that is lethal to the cancer cells. PDT can also harm the tumor's blood vessels, making it difficult for the tumor to grow and spread. Additionally, it can activate the immune system to attack the cancer cells in other parts of the body.

SIDE EFFECTS OF PDT

PDT may cause some side effects, such as burns, swelling, pain, and scarring in the treatment area, as well as coughing, stomach pain, and shortness of breath, depending on the location of the treatment. A specific type of photosensitizer, called porfimer sodium, can make the skin and eyes sensitive to light for up to six weeks after treatment, which requires avoiding bright light. ECP, another type of therapy, can cause low blood pressure, faster-than-normal heart rate, anemia, and low blood platelet count, but these side effects usually improve after treatment.

RADIOTHERAPY

Radiation therapy, also known as radiotherapy, is a treatment for cancer that utilizes high doses of radiation to eliminate cancer cells and decrease tumor size. Radiation is also used in x-rays to view the inside of the body, such as in the case of x-rays of broken bones or teeth, but at lower doses.

HOW RADIOTHERAPY WORKS.

Radiation therapy operates against cancer by causing DNA damage to cancer cells or slowing their growth at high doses. Cancer cells with irreparable DNA damage stop dividing or die and are subsequently broken down and removed by the body. It typically takes several days or weeks of treatment for DNA to be damaged enough for cancer cells to begin dying, and they continue to die for weeks or months after treatment is completed.

TYPES OF CANCER THAT ARE TREATED WITH RADIOTHERAPY.

Radiation therapy is used to treat many types of cancer, such as with external beam radiation therapy. Brachytherapy is most commonly used to treat cancers in the head and neck, breast, cervix, prostate, and eye. In addition, a systemic radiation therapy known as radioactive iodine (I-131) is typically used to treat certain types of thyroid cancer, while targeted radionuclide therapy is used to treat patients with advanced prostate cancer or gastroenteropancreatic neuroendocrine tumor (GEP-NET), also known as molecular radiotherapy. Radiopharmaceuticals are drugs that can deliver radiation therapy directly and specifically to cancer cells.

STEM CELL TRANSPLANT.

Stem cell transplants are medical procedures that aim to restore blood-forming stem cells in individuals whose own stem cells have been damaged or destroyed by high doses of chemotherapy or radiation therapy used in the treatment of certain cancers. Blood-forming stem cells play a crucial role in the growth of different types of blood cells, such as white blood cells, red blood cells, and platelets, all of which are necessary for maintaining good health.

HOW STEM CELL TRANSPLANT WORK

Although stem cell transplants do not usually work directly against cancer, they help to restore the body's ability to produce stem cells after intensive radiation therapy, chemotherapy, or both. In some cases, such as in multiple myeloma and some types of leukemia, stem cell transplants can work directly against cancer through a process known as graft-versus-tumor, where white blood cells from the donor attack any remaining cancer cells in the recipient's body, improving the success of treatment.

SIDE EFFECTS OF STEM CELL TRANSPLANT

Stem cell transplants can cause side effects due to the high doses of cancer treatment received before the transplant, including an increased risk of infection and bleeding. Additionally, those who receive an allogeneic transplant may develop graft-versus-host disease, a serious condition where the donor's white blood cells attack the recipient's body, potentially causing damage to various organs. The likelihood of developing this condition can be reduced by finding a donor with a closer match to the recipient's stem cells, and by administering drugs to suppress the immune system. It's important to discuss potential side effects and how to manage them with a healthcare provider.

SURGERY

When cancer is treated with surgery, a surgeon will use scalpels and other sharp tools to remove cancer from the body. Anesthesia is used to prevent the patient from feeling pain during the procedure, and there are three types of anesthesia: local, regional, and general. In addition to traditional surgery with scalpels, other techniques like cryosurgery, lasers, hyperthermia, and photodynamic therapy can be used to treat cancer.

TYPE OF CANCER THAT IS TREATED WITH SURGERY

Surgery is most effective for solid tumors that are contained in one area and are not used for blood cancers or cancers that have spread. Depending on the type and stage of cancer, surgery can be used to remove the entire tumor, debulk a tumor, or ease cancer symptoms.

SIDE EFFECTS OF SURGERY

Although surgeons are highly trained to prevent problems during surgery, there are risks involved such as pain, infection, bleeding, and damage to nearby tissues. Patients should talk to their doctor about the possible risks before undergoing surgery.

TARGETED THERAPY

Targeted therapy is a cancer treatment that focuses on the proteins responsible for the growth, division, and spread of cancer cells. Unlike chemotherapy, which attacks all fast-growing cells, targeted therapy is specific to cancer cells. There are various ways in which targeted therapy works, including boosting the immune system, interrupting signals that cause uncontrolled growth, preventing the formation of blood vessels, delivering cell-killing substances to cancer cells, causing cancer cell death, and starving cancer of hormones it needs to grow.

SIDE EFFECTS OF TARGETED THERAPY

Although initially believed to be less toxic than chemotherapy, targeted therapy can still have side effects such as diarrhea, liver problems, high blood pressure, fatigue, mouth sores, and skin problems. However, medications are available to prevent or treat these side effects, and they usually subside once the treatment ends.